Blood Pressure Solutions

MW01296105

Blood Pressure: The Ultimate Guide to Lowering Your Blood Pressure Naturally with Natural Remedies without medication in 90 days.

Table of Contents

Introduction

Thank you for downloading *Blood Pressure Solutions: Blood Pressure: The Ultimate Guide to Lowering Your Blood Pressure Naturally with Natural Remedies without medication in 90 days!*

You're going to find so much information in this book that will completely change your mind about being diagnosed with hypertension and how to handle it. In most cases, hypertension can easily be managed with a change in diet and taking a few extra supplements every day, as well as monitoring by your doctor to make sure progress is being made. A diagnosis of hypertension is not the end of the world, nor is it the end of your life.

You'll find information pertaining to how you can lead a healthier life through exercise and diet when you have hypertension, as well as what herbs and supplements you can take in order to lower your blood pressure. If you're not sure how you're progressing, you'll also figure out how to measure your blood pressure at home accurately so that you can monitor your own progress.

There's a ton of useful information you'll find in this book, so I encourage you to keep reading!

This document is geared towards providing exact and reliable information in regards to the topic and issue covered. The publication is sold with the idea that the publisher is not required to render accounting, officially permitted, or otherwise, qualified services. If advice is necessary, legal or professional, a practiced individual in the profession should be ordered.

- From a Declaration of Principles which was accepted and approved equally by a Committee of the American Bar Association and a Committee of Publishers and Associations.

The information provided herein is stated to be truthful and consistent, in that any liability, in terms of inattention or otherwise, by any usage or abuse of any policies, processes, or directions contained within is the solitary and utter responsibility of the recipient reader. Under no circumstances will any legal responsibility or blame be held against the publisher for any reparation, damages, or

Chapter One – Understanding High Blood Pressure

You've just been to the doctor due to some disturbing symptoms, or maybe it was for something that you thought was simple, and know you've been diagnosed with high blood pressure. Hypertension, or high blood pressure, is not very uncommon in the United States anymore, and there seem to be one of two reactions that people have to being diagnosed with it. Some people are shocked they have it and want to find out whatever they can about the disease to determine how they can cure themselves of it, while others have heard of it so often they don't think of it as a threat to their health.

Well, hypertension is a threat to your health, and a serious one, at that. Since you're reading this book, I'm going to assume you're someone who wants to understand what they've been diagnosed with, and how they can overcome it.

So without further delay, let's get started with what hypertension is!

What is Blood Pressure?

Your blood pressure is the force at which your blood pushes against the walls of your arteries while your heart is pumping. When you have hypertension, this is when that force is too high. Your doctor will check your blood pressure with a gauge, electronic sensor, or a stethoscope. With this equipment, they will measure your systolic pressure, which is the blood pressure when your heart is beating and pumping blood, and your diastolic pressure, which is when your heart is at rest between beats. These two numbers make up your blood pressure reading, with your systolic pressure being first and your diastolic pressure being the second number.

Normal blood pressure for an adult is defined as being a systolic pressure that is below 120/80. It's normal for your blood pressure to change throughout your day, such as when you wake up when you're sleeping, and when you're nervous or excited about something. When you're active, it's normal for your blood pressure levels to rise, and when you stop being activity, your blood pressure ought to return to its normal rate.

Blood pressure will normally increase as you get older and if you gain weight. A newborn baby will have a low blood pressure number that's considered normal, while an older teen will have a number similar to an adult.

An abnormal blood pressure is someone who has a reading over 120/80.

While blood pressure increases seen in those who are prehypertension are less than those who are diagnosed with hypertension, prehypertension is able to progress into hypertension and should be taken seriously. Over time, a consistently high blood press will damage and weaken your blood vessels, which can lead to some serious complications.

There are two main types of hypertension. These are primary and secondary hypertension.

Primary hypertension is the most common form of hypertension. This form tends to develop over the years as you age. Secondary hypertension is caused by a separate medical condition or use of a medication. This type will usually resolve after the cause has been treated or removed.

What are the causes of high blood pressure?

Changes due to your genetics or your environment can cause hypertension, including changes in your salt balances and kidneys, your sympathetic nervous system, your renin-angiotensin-aldosterone system, and your blood vessel structure and its health.

Changes in your kidneys can cause hypertension. The kidneys tend to regulate your body's salt levels by retaining water and sodium while excreting potassium. Imbalances in your kidney function can expand your blood's volume, which can cause hypertension.

The renin-angiotensin-aldosterone system is what makes the aldosterone and angiotensin hormones. Aldosterone controls how your kidneys balance the fluids and salt levels, and angiotensin constricts your blood vessels. Increased aldosterone in your system or activity can change your kidney function, leading to hypertension due to high blood volumes.

Changes in your sympathetic nervous system can also cause hypertension. This system has imperative functions in regulating your blood pressure, including your actual blood pressure, heart rate, and your breathing rate. Researches are still investigating into whether or not imbalances in this system are the cause of hypertension.

In addition, changes in your actual blood vessel structure and function can also cause hypertension. Changes in both the small and large arteries can contribute to hypertension. The angiotensin pathway and your immune system can stiffen the small and large arteries, which will affect your blood pressure levels.

There can also be genetic causes of hypertension. Much of the knowledge about hypertension has been derived from genetic studies of the diseases. Hypertension tends to run in families. Years of research has identified a few genes and other mutations that are associated with the condition. However, these known genetic factors tend to account for only two to three percent of all cases of the condition. Emerging research suggests some DNA changes in the course of fetal development can also cause the growth of hypertension later on in your life.

An unhealthy lifestyle, such as a high amount of sodium intake, as well as sodium sensitivity, can cause hypertension. Also, drinking excessive amounts of alcohol and smoking are contributing factors. Lack of exercise that leads to obesity is also another factor that can contribute to hypertension, and some medications have been shown to be conducive to causing this illness.

Who is at a risk of developing high BP?

There are numerous different causes of hypertension, but there are some risk factors that you should be aware of.

First, age is the most common risk factor. As you age, your risk of developing hypertension increases greatly. Around sixty-five percent of Americans who are over the age of sixty have hypertension. However, the risk for this ailment is rising for children and teens due to the rise in the number of overweight children and teens.

Second, your ethnicity can be another contributing factor. Hypertension is more common in African Americans than in Hispanic American or Caucasian adults. Compared to these ethnic groups, African Americans tend to have hypertension earlier on in life, have a higher blood pressure number, and are less likely to achieve their goals for hypertension treatments.

Men are more likely than women to develop hypertension before the age of fifty-five. However, after the age of fifty-five, women are more likely than men to develop it if they have not already.

The most important factor is a family history of hypertension. If you have any close relatives, such as parents or grandparents, who have the disorder, then you are at a higher risk of developing hypertension. Genetics plays a large role in the development of this disease, so you should be checked out often by a doctor if you have a family history of it.

What are the side effects of hypertension?

While hypertension might not seem like the most frightening diagnosis at first, there are some serious side effects that should be considered.

First and foremost, aneurysms are a serious side effect of hypertension. This is when there is an abnormal bulge in the wall of one of your arteries. Aneurysms occur and grow for years without causing symptoms or signs until they finally rupture, grow large enough to press on a nearby body part, or block the blood flow. The symptoms and signs that develop will depend on the location of the aneurysms, but they are very life threatening.

Second, chronic kidney disease is another disease caused by hypertension and the two feed on one another. As the blood vessels in the kidneys narrow, hypertension becomes worse. This can eventually lead to kidney failure.

The next side effect is cognitive changes. Research has shown that, over time, hypertension can lead to cognitive changes. Symptoms and signs will include difficulty finding words, memory loss, and losing focus while you're having a conversation.

You can also experience damage to your eyes. This occurs because the blood vessels in the eyes will bleed or burst due to the pressure. The signs and symptoms include changes in vision and, eventually, blindness.

Of course, most people associate hypertension with heart attacks, which is absolutely true. When the flow of oxygenated blood to a section of your heart muscle is suddenly blocked and it doesn't get enough oxygen, you experience a heart attack. The most common symptoms are upper body discomfort, chest pain and discomfort, and shortness of breath.

Related to heart attacks is heart failure. When the heart is not able to pump enough blood to meet your body's demands, you go through heart failure. The symptoms of this include feeling tired, shortness of breath and trouble breathing, and swelling of your legs, ankles, feet, veins in your neck, and your abdomen.

Peripheral artery disease is a disease where plaque builds up in your leg arteries and affects the blood flow to your legs. When you have symptoms of this, the most common ones are cramping, pain, aching, numbness, heaviness of your feet, legs, and behind after you walk or climb stairs.

Finally, stroke is another side effect of untreated hypertension. When the flow of oxygenated blood to portions of your brain is blocked, stroke happens. The symptoms include an abrupt start of feebleness, paralysis of your legs, face, or arms, and trouble speaking or seeing.

What are the benefits of lowering high BP?

Of course, the main benefits of lowering your blood pressure is lowering your risk for developing all of the aforementioned ailments.

You'll be able to avoid heart complications. Hypertension puts a strain on the heart, which increases your risk of peripheral artery disease, angina, heart attack, coronary artery disease, and heart failure. Damaged arteries that result in hypertension collect plaque become hardened, and then narrow. Over time, the heart will become damaged and it will enlarge. The damage to your heart cannot be undone. Lowering your blood pressure to a normal level will prevent any future damage and help mitigate any previous damage by allowing your heart to work under the best conditions.

You will also avoid the risk of stroke. Hypertension puts a strain on the blood vessels throughout your entire body. When a blood vessel in your brain becomes blocked by a clot or bursts, a stroke occurs. Chronic hypertension is a risk factor for hemorrhage stroke, and the potential damage caused by hypertension contributes to ischemic stroke. Getting your hypertension under control can reduce your risk of developing a stroke, but it will not reduce the complications associated with a stroke.

You'll also improve your vision if you get your hypertension under control. Hypertension is known to put a strain on the eyes. The damage to your vision caused by hypertension will build up over time. Lowering your blood pressure to a normal level will reduce the strain that's put on your optic nerve, which is the nerve that is responsible for your ability to see. Uncontrolled hypertension can lead to hypertensive retinopathy, which is a disease that affects your eye's retina.

Lastly, you'll boost your kidney health. Your kidneys produce the hormone that helps regulate your blood pressure. Hypertension will damage your kidneys, and once they've been damaged, they will no longer help regulate your blood pressure. Lowering your blood pressure prevents this vicious cycle from occurring, and lowers your risk for total kidney failure.

Know how to measure your own blood pressure.

Knowing how to measure your own blood pressure at home can literally mean the difference between life and death. Depending on your condition, your doctor may instruct you to take your pulse regularly and determine what your blood pressure is. This will help you figure out if what you're experiencing is a true emergency or not.

So, before you check your blood pressure, there are a few things you need to do. First, you need to find a quiet space to do this. You'll need to listen for your heartbeat. Second, make sure you're comfortable and relaxed, and that you've recently emptied your bladder. Yes, your bladder being full can affect your reading. Third, you have to roll up the sleeve on your arm and remove any tight-sleeved clothing. Lastly, rest in a chair for five to ten minutes. Your arm needs to rest comfortably at your heart's level. Make sure that you're sitting with good posture, and you have your back against the chair and your legs uncrossed. Place your forearms on the table in front of you with the palm of your hand facing up.

To check your blood pressure, follow these steps.

1. Locate your pulse. You can do this by lightly pressing your index finger and your middle finger tightly to the inside center of your inner elbow. If you can't find your pulse, then put the head of a stethoscope or an arm cuff in the same general region.

2. Secure the cuff. Thread your cuff end through the metal loop and slide it onto your arm, making sure the stethoscope is over the artery. The cuff can be marked with an arrow to show you the location of the stethoscope head. The lower edge of the cuff needs to be about an inch above the inner area of your elbow. Use the fabric fastener to make it snug, but don't make it too tight. Put the stethoscope in your ears and tilt the ear piece a bit forward to get a good sound.

3. Inflate and deflate your cuff.

   a. If you're using a manual one, hold the pressure gauge in your left hand and the bulb in your right hand. Close the airflow valve by turning the screw clockwise.

b. Inflate by squeezing the bulb with your right hand. You'll probably hear your pulse at this point.

c. Watch the gauge and keep inflating until it reaches thirty points above your expected systolic pressure. You shouldn't hear your pulses at this point.

d. Keep your eyes on the gauge and slowly release the pressure in the cuff by opening the airflow valve the opposite direction you used to close it. The gauge should fall just two to three points with every heartbeat.

e. Listen carefully for your first pulse beat. As soon as you hear that, note the reading on the gauge. This is your systolic pressure.

f. Continue to deflate the cuff. Listen until the sound disappears. As soon as you can't hear it any longer, note the reading on the gauge. That is your diastolic pressure.

g. Let the cuff completely deflate.

4. Record your blood pressure. You should record the date, time, and the two numbers so that you can keep track of your blood pressure. Do this as often as your doctor recommends.

Chapter Two – Lifestyle Changes You Can Make to Lower Your Blood Pressure

There are numerous lifestyle changes you can make in order to lower your blood pressure and become healthy again.

Healthy Eating

To help treat your hypertension, health care providers recommend that you reduce your salt and sodium intake, increase your potassium intake, and eat foods that are healthy for your heart.

To limit sodium and salt, try choosing and preparing foods naturally lower in these two components. Try to use some no added salt and low sodium foods and seasonings when you're cooking. Food labels will let you know what you should know about choosing foods that are lower in sodium. Attempt to eat no more than 2,300mg of sodium per day. If you have hypertension, you might need to limit your sodium consumption even greater.

Your health care provider might recommend the DASH Diet. You'll learn more about this eating plan later on in the book in the healthy eating chapter.

Being Physically Active

Routine physical activity could lower your blood pressure and reduce your risk for many other disease and complications. Talk with a doctor about starting an exercise plan. Ask them how much and how often you should engage in physical activity as everyone has to start at a different and safe level.

You should try to participate in moderate to intense aerobic exercises around two hours a week. Aerobic exercise is brisk walking, playing tennis, or any other activity that gets your heart pumping.

You'll learn more about exercise in the following chapters.

Maintaining a Healthy Weight

Staying at a healthy weight will help you control your hypertension and reduce your risk for many other heath complications. If you've been told you're overweight or obese by a healthcare provider, try to lose weight. A loss of just three to five percent will lessen your risk of developing heart problems. A greater amount of weight loss can improve your blood pressure readings, lower your LDL cholesterol, and increase your HDL cholesterol.

Limiting Alcohol Intake

You should limit your alcohol intake because too much alcohol will increase your blood pressure and your triglyceride levels. This is a type of fat that's found in the blood. Alcohol will also add some extra calories, which can contribute to weight gain. Men shouldn't have any more than two drinks in a day while women ought to only have one drink in a day.

Managing and Coping With Stress

Learning how to relax, cope with stress, and cope with your difficulties can mend your physical and your emotional health. This will help lower your blood pressure. Stress management techniques will be discussed further in future chapters of this book.

Medicines

Blood pressure medications work in different ways to slow down or stop some of your body's functions that might be causing hypertension. Medications that lower hypertension include:

- Diuretics: These flush out excess sodium from your body through increased urination. Be sure you drink a lot of water if you take these!

- Beta Blockers: These help the heart beat slower and with less force so that your heart pumps a lesser amount of blood through the blood vessels.

- ACE Inhibitors: These block the conversion of Angiotensin I to Angiotensin II, which is what causes hypertension.

- ARBs: These block the angiotensin II hormone from reacting with the receptors in the blood vessels.

- Calcium Channel Blockers: These keep calcium from entering the muscle cells of the heart and blood vessels.

- Alpha Blockers: These reduce the nerve impulses that tighten your blood vessels.

- Alpha-Beta Blockers: These reduce the nerve impulses just like Alpha Blockers, but these slow down the heartbeat.

- Central Acting Agents: These act on the brain in order to reduce the nerve signals that narrow the blood vessels.

- Vasodilators: these relax the muscles in the blood vessel walls, which will lower blood pressure.

Now that you know about the different lifestyle changes let's go over them in more detail in the following chapters.

Chapter Three – Dietary Changes That Will Combat High Blood Pressure

Changing your diet is one of the best ways to alleviate the symptoms of almost any disease in the body, and hypertension is not an exception. There are many ways that you can change your diet in order to combat your hypertension, so let's take a look at them in this first section,

and then we'll talk more about some of the foods you should be eating.

General Dietary Changes

First and foremost, you should be cooking as much as you can at home. Cooking at home is an imperative part of lowering your blood pressure, which is why those who created the DASH diet recommend that you do this. This means you're keeping your diet as unprocessed as you can, which means consuming fewer things that come in a package, avoiding restaurant and takeout foods, and limiting your fast food considerably. Making your own homemade meals from nutrient-dense, fresh ingredients allows you to lower your sugar and sodium consumption while you boost your intake of powerful nutrients such as antioxidants, potassium, and fiber, all of which can help you lower your blood pressure.

Second, you'll want to increase your fiber consumption. Consuming enough fiber has shown to help prevent high blood pressure, plus it manages your appetite and helps you avoid that blood sugar roller coaster of cravings, fatigue, bad digestion, and many other health complications. Fiber is able to be found in almost all unprocessed plant foods, so eating fresh vegetables will not only help you adopt a high-fiber diet, but they will also help you lower your blood pressure. Foods high in fiber also help you reduce your risk of high triglycerides, diabetes, high cholesterol, weight gain, and digestive complications.

You'll also want to consider lowering your sodium consumption overall. A low sodium diet is the most recommended way to controlling your blood pressure levels because high amounts of sodium have been proven to worsen hypertension by impacting your fluid retention levels and how your arteries dilate.

Sodium is an electrolyte that's balanced by the other electrolytes in your body, such as magnesium and potassium, in order to keep your blood pressure at a healthy rate. The problem is most people who are eating the standard American diet consume way too much sodium and a lot less magnesium and potassium than they need, which leads to an electrolyte imbalance.

In addition to lowering your sodium levels, you'll want to boost your potassium intake. A low potassium, high sodium diet is one of the main contributors to hypertension and other cardiovascular diseases. Potassium is found in foods such as sweet potatoes, green vegetables, bananas, organic dairy products, avocados, and beans, and is the third most abundant mineral in your body. It's necessary to interact with sodium in order to perform many different functions.

Potassium naturally increases the sodium excretion and is found in all your cells because it plays a role in regulating your nerve impulses, heartbeat rhythms, digestive health, and muscle contractions. Low potassium will raise the fluid retention in your body, as well as elevate your blood pressure by interfering with your heart rate and the narrowing of your arteries.

Another imperative factor to keep in mind is how hydrated you are. Drinking plenty of water throughout the day is important for preventing an imbalance in fluids, dehydrations, fatigue, and cravings. Drink more fresh water in place of thing such as soda, juice, and sweetened tea and coffee. Be sure to have around eight eight-ounce glasses of water per day.

Lastly, practice portion control at your meals and snack times. There isn't any reason to get overwhelmed and be afraid that you'll never be able to eat your favorite snacks or foods again. Focus on filling up on the things that are healthy first so that you're less likely to crave the unhealthy things. Watch your portions and practice mindful eating to be sure your body gets what it craves to feel good but not too much that makes you feel weighed down.

Dietary Electrolytes

There are seven main electrolytes in the body. These are sodium, chloride, potassium, magnesium, calcium, phosphate, and bicarbonate. Together, these seven electrolytes keep your body healthy and running smoothly. When they become imbalanced, you experience diseases, such as hypertension.

Sodium

Sodium is an essential electrolyte for people that control the total amount of water that's in your body. It's imperative for regulating your blood volume and maintaining your nerve and muscle function. It's a major positively charged ion outside the body's cells and is mostly found in your blood plasma, blood, and lymph fluids. This makes one-half the electrical pump that keeps your electrolytes in balance between the intracellular and extracellular environments.

An excess of sodium is known as hypernatremia and usually comes from dehydration. This leads to lethargy, weakness, and sometimes seizures and coma, in the more severe cases. Having too little sodium in the body is known as hyponatremia, and is the most common electrolyte disorder in the United States. It causes symptoms such as confusion, headache, hallucinations, fatigue, and muscle spasms.

Most people who have hypertension have an excess of sodium, so this is one you most likely won't need to supplement.

Chloride

This is the major negatively charged ion electrolyte that is usually found in the extracellular fluid. It works closely with the sodium in your body to maintain the proper amount of pressure on the numerous fluid compartments of your body, such as in your blood, cells, and the fluid between your cells.

It's also extremely important for maintaining the proper acidity in your body, passively balance the positive ions in your blood, organs, and tissue.

Just like sodium, most chloride is obtained through consuming salt. Chloride toxicity and deficiencies are rare, but they could occur because of another electrolyte being out of balance. Symptoms include respiratory difficulties and a pH imbalance.

Potassium

Where sodium is usually found outside of the cell, potassium is the major electrolyte found inside the cells and is imperative for regulating your muscle function and your heartbeat. It creates the other half of the electrical pump that keeps your electrolytes in balance and lets conductivity occur between cells, making potassium the critical part of neuron transmission.

Milk, meat, fruits, and vegetables have a lot of potassium in them, but the average person still doesn't get enough in their diet. The proper balance of potassium and sodium in the body is imperative to maintaining your health, but people often skip on the natural vegetables and fruits that are full of potassium in favor of foods that are higher in sodium. What's worse is the imbalance of potassium and sodium is what causes hypertension, stroke, and heart disease.

Mostly, potassium toxicity in the body is pretty rare, but it's fatal if it's not treated quickly because it causes paralysis of the lungs, irregular heartbeat, and cardiac arrest. An overdose is so dangerous that it's deliberately used for lethal injection in the United States using a mixture of potassium chloride. However, a deficiency in the electrolyte is common and is often caused by a loss of water due to severe diarrhea or vomiting. Minor cases have lesser symptoms such as cramping and muscle weakness; however, severe cases are deadly and should be treated immediately.

If you have hypertension, be sure to have your potassium levels checked to make sure you are not deficient in this electrolyte, as it could very well be the cause of your hypertension, and it's easily amended.

Magnesium

If you take into consideration just how critical it is to life on this planet, magnesium is probably the most under-appreciated mineral. Not only is this mineral necessary for over three hundred biochemical reactions in your body, but it also has an imperative role in the synthesis of RNA and DNA, essential to each and every cell of every known living organism on this planet. The fourth most prevalent mineral in our bodies, magnesium, allows your body to maintain normal muscle and nerve function, boost your immune system, maintains your heart rate at a stable level, stabilizes your blood glucose and promotes the formation of teeth and bones. Spices, nuts, leafy green vegetables, tea, and coffee are all good sources of this mineral.

Hypermagnesemia or high levels of this mineral in the body is pretty rare due to the body being very efficient at getting rid of any excess, making it hard to consume too much through your diet. Magnesium toxicity could occur in the case of excessive supplementation or kidney failure, and could lead to vomiting, nausea, impaired breathing, and an irregular heartbeat. A magnesium deficiency is most commonly found on alcoholics due to the kidneys excreting around 260% more magnesium than they usually do after you've consumed alcohol, but the condition is caused by malnutrition, too. Symptoms are convulsions, fatigue, numbness, and muscle spasms.

Calcium

Calcium is not only good for the formation of teeth and bones, but it's also imperative for the transmission of nerve signals, muscle contractions, and blood clotting. Being the most abundant mineral in the body, about ninety-nine percent of calcium is found in your skeletal structure, but your body also needs it in the bloodstream and other cells. If there isn't enough calcium in the blood, it's taken from the bones to supplement the deficiency. When this is left unchecked, the lack of calcium will lead to osteoporosis.

The recommended amount of calcium for an adult is anywhere from 1000-1,500mg per day to maintain the proper amount in your bloodstream and avoid weakening your bones. Too much calcium is very uncommon, but can come from an excessive consumption of foods high in calcium, bone diseases, or extreme inactivity. Symptoms can include digestive upset in minor cases, or brain dysfunction, death, or coma in some extreme cases. Moderate cases might not cause immediate symptoms, but over time, it will affect the brain, leading to memory loss, delirium, and depression. Severe cases can lead to seizures, muscle spasms, and abnormal heart rates.

Phosphate

Phosphorous is second to calcium when it comes to being the most abundant mineral in the body, eighty-five percent of which is found in your bones. The phosphate works closely with the calcium in order to strengthen the teeth and bones, but it's also essential to energy production in your cells, necessary for tissue growth and repair, and is a huge building block for all the cell membranes and your DNA.

Most people obtain the right amount of phosphorus through what they eat, but high levels are not uncommon and generally indicate a calcium deficiency or kidney disease. Increased phosphate in your body has also been linked with a greater risk of heart disease. Hypophosphatemia is a lot less common but happens more frequently with those who have Crohn's disease or are alcoholics. Symptoms of this condition include weakened bones, joint pain, irregular breathing, and fatigue.

Bicarbonate

Your body relies on a sophisticated buffering system in order to maintain the proper pH levels. The lungs regulate the amount of carbon dioxide in your body, most of which is combined with water and made into carbonic acid. This acid is quickly converted into bicarbonate, which is the key element in the pH buffer.

When acids build up through a metabolic process or a production of lactic acid in the muscles, the kidneys will release bicarbonate to counteract the higher level of acid in the body. If the body is too base, the kidneys will lessen the amount of bicarbonate and increase acidity. Without this system in place, rapid changes in pH balance might cause serious complications in the body such as damaging sensitive tissue around the nervous system. This bicarbonate cushion is one of the main reasons your body is able to maintain homeostasis and function correctly.

The bottom line is that you need to have all your electrolyte levels tested routinely to make sure they are of the proper amount. If one of them seems low, discuss your options with a doctor to see what you can do about getting it back into balance.

What's the best diet plan to follow for hypertension?

The DASH diet is the most recommended diet by doctors out there for those who have hypertension. There are two versions of the DASH diet. Both of them include plenty of fruits, whole grains, vegetables, and low-fat dairy products. The DASH diet also includes poultry, fish, legume, and encourages you to consume a small amount of nuts and seeds a few times a week.

Yu can consume sweet, red meat and fat in small amounts. The DASH diet is a diet that is low in saturated fat, total fat, and cholesterol.

Let's take a look at the recommended servings from every food group for a 2,000 calorie DASH diet plan.

Grains 6-8 Servings per Day

Grains are cereal, bread, pasta, and rice. Examples of a serving of grains are a slice of whole-wheat bread, an ounce of dry cereal, or half a cup of cooked cereal, pasta, or rice.

You should focus on whole grains because they have more nutrients and fiber than refined grains. For example, use whole wheat pasta rather than regular pasta, brown rice rather than white rice, and whole grain bread rather than white bread. Search for products that are labeled 100% whole grain or 100% whole wheat. Naturally low in fat, grains should be kept this way by avoiding any cream, butter, or cheese sauces.

Vegetables 4-5 Servings per Day

Broccoli, tomatoes, carrots, greens, sweet potatoes, and many other vegetables are packed full of vitamins, fiber, and minerals that you need, such as magnesium and potassium. Examples of a serving include a cup of leafy green vegetables or half a cup of cooked or raw vegetables.

Don't think of your vegetables as being good for just side dishes. A hearty blend of vegetables that are served with some whole-wheat noodles or over some whole-grain rice is definitely a main dish for a meal. Fresh and frozen vegetables are also good choices. When you're purchasing frozen or canned vegetables, choose the ones that do not have any added salt or are labeled as low sodium.

To increase the number of daily servings you fit in, get a little creative. Stir-fries can be doubled up on the vegetables and halved with the amount of meat they contain.

Fruits 4-5 Servings per Day

Most fruits need very little if any, preparation in order to become a healthy snack or meal.

Just like vegetables, they're packed with potassium, magnesium, and fiber, as well as being low in fat. Coconuts are an exception to the rule. Examples of a serving include a medium fruit, half a cup of fresh, canned, or frozen fruit, or four ounces of juice.

You could try having a whole fruit as a snack and one at a meal, and then round your day with some dessert of low-fat yogurt and fresh fruits. You should leave on the edible peels whenever you can. The peels of pears, apples, and most fruits that have pits will add an interesting texture to your recipes, and they contain healthy fiber and nutrients.

Keep in mind that citrus juices and fruits, such as grapefruit, will interact with certain medications, so check with a pharmacist or doctor to see if they're alright for you. If you choose some canned fruit or juices, be sure there isn't any added sugar.

Dairy 2-3 Servings per Day

Yogurt, milk, cheese and many other dairy products are a major source of vitamin D, calcium, and protein. However, the key is to be sure that you choose dairy products that are low in fat or fat-free because they can be a major source of dietary fat, and most of it will be saturated. Examples of a serving include a cup of skim or one percent milk, a cup of low-fat yogurt, or one and a half ounces of part-skim cheese.

Fat-free and low-fat frozen yogurt will help boost the amount of dairy products you consume while offering you a dessert option. Add some fruit for a healthy twist. If you have trouble with dairy products due to a lactose intolerance, choose some lactose-free items or consider taking an over-the-counter medication, such as Lactaid, that will reduce or prevent the symptoms of lactose intolerance.

You should be sure to go easy on the regular and fat-free cheeses because they are usually high in sodium.

Poultry, Lean Meat, and Fish 6 Servings or Less per Day

Meat is a rich source of B vitamins, protein, zinc, and iron. Choose the lean varieties and try to go for no more than six ounces a day. Cutting back on how much meat you consume will leave you more room to consume more vegetables.

Trim away the skin and the fat from the meat and poultry and bake, grill, or broil rather than frying the meat in fat. Eat the heart-healthy fish, such as herring, salmon, and tuna. These types are high in omega-3 fatty acids, which will help lower your cholesterol levels.

Seeds, Nuts, and Legumes 4-5 Servings per Week

Sunflower seeds, almonds, kidney beans, lentils, peas, and other foods in this family are an excellent source of potassium, magnesium, and protein. They are also full of phytochemicals and fiber, which are plant compounds that can protect you against some cardiovascular diseases and cancer.

Serving sizes should be small and are intended to be eaten only a few times a week due to these foods being high in calories. Examples of a serving include a third of a cup of nuts, two tablespoons of seeds, or half a cup of cooked peas or beans.

Nuts tend to get a bad reputation due to their high fat content, but they have the healthy kinds of fat. They're high in calories, though, so eat them sparingly. Try adding them to salads, stir-fries, and cereals.

Soybean based products, such as tempeh and tofu, are a good alternative to meat because they have all the amino acids your body needs in order to make a complete protein, just like meat does.

Oils and Fats 2-3 Servings per Day

Fat allows your body to absorb essential nutrients and vitamins, and they keep your immune system healthy. However, too much fat will increase your risk for diabetes, heart disease, and obesity. The DASH diet is meant to help balance your diet by limiting your total fat to less than thirty percent of your daily calories, with a focus on the monounsaturated fats that are healthier.

Examples of a serving of fat include a teaspoon of soft margarine, two tablespoons of salad dressing, and a tablespoon of mayonnaise.

The main dietary culprits that increase your risk of coronary artery disease are trans-fat and saturated fat. DASH helps keep the daily saturated fat intake to less than six percent of your total calories by limiting the consumption of butter, meat, cheese, cream, whole milk, and eggs.

You want to avoid trans-fat, which is commonly found in processed foods like baked goods, crackers, and fried foods. Be sure you read the food labels on salad dressing and margarine so that you can choose the ones that are the lowest in saturated fat and free from trans-fat.

Desserts or Sweets 5 Servings or Less per Week

You don't need to get rid of dessert entirely while you're following the DASH diet, but you need to go easy on them. An example of one serving includes one tablespoon of sugar, a tablespoon of jam or jelly, half a cup of sorbet, or a cup of lemonade.

When you consume sweets, choose ones that are low-fat or fat-free, such as fruit ices, sorbets, jelly beans, graham crackers, low-fat cookies, or hard candy.

Artificial sweeteners can help curb that sweet tooth while sparing you the consumption of sugar. However, you still have to use them sensibly. It's okay to swap in a diet coke for a regular one, but not in place of a more nutritious beverage, such as water.

Be sure to cut back on the added sugar, which doesn't have any nutritional value and packs on the calories.

Now that you know how to eat healthier let's take a look at how you can use exercise to lose weight and lower your blood pressure.

Chapter Four – Exercise Programs to Lose Weight and Lower Blood Pressure

Everyone needs to get regular exercise in order to improve their fitness and health. Those who are not physically active are a lot more likely to develop health complications. Even moderately intense activities, such as biking or brisk

walking, is beneficial when it's done regularly for thirty minutes or longer at least five days a week. Lack of physical exercise increases your risk of stroke and heart attack and contributes to obesity. Regular physical activity will help reduce your blood pressure, reduce your stress, and control your weight.

Finding the Time

Most people's argument for not exercising is

they can't seem to find the time to do it. When it comes to physical activity, you just need to get moving! Find some ways you can enjoy the benefits as you gradually increase your activity levels.

First, don't be afraid to get more active. If you've not been active for quite a bit of time, or if you're beginning a new exercise or activity program, then take it slowly. Consult your doctor if you have cardiovascular disease or another pre-existing condition. It's better to begin slowly with something that you like, such as taking walks or riding a bicycle. Scientific evidence strongly suggests that physical activity is safe for just about everyone. In addition, the health benefits of physical activity far outweigh any risks.

If you love going outside, combine it with some physical activity and enjoy the scenery as you're jogging or walking. If you love to listen to some audiobooks, then enjoy them while you're on a treadmill.

Some activities that are overall beneficial when they're done on a regular basis are walking, hiking, stair-climbing, running, jogging, bicycling, swimming rowing, fitness classes, team sports, fitness games, and dance classes.

You should also make sure that you mix it up from time to time. A variety of activities will help you stay interested and motivated in what you're doing. When you include flexibility and strength goals, you help reduce your chance of injury so that you can maintain a good level of heart-healthy fitness for years to come.

Understand Moderation

If you get hurt right at the beginning, you're less likely to keep motivated. Focus on performing an activity that will get your heart rate up to a moderate level. Being physically active regularly for a longer period of time or at a greater intensity will help you benefit more.

However, don't overdo it. Too much exercise will give you sore muscles and increase your risk of injury.

Reward Yourself

You can do this by making your exercise social time. Walk with a friend, neighbor or a spouse. Take an exercise challenge. Connect with others who are like you and can keep you focused and motivated to do more.

In addition, reward yourself with something that supports your goal. Pay yourself by setting aside a small amount of money every time you work out. After a month, invest that payment in something that inspires you to keep working out, like some new music to enjoy as you jog or a new workout shirt.

Celebrate all your milestones. Fitness is a regular part of life, or it should be, so find some ways to savor that success. Log workout times or distances and write yourself a congratulation note when you've achieved a milestone, or get a massage every one hundred miles. Use whatever healthy incentive you can to keep you motivated, but don't use food!

Healthy Exercise Tips

There are some things that you should remember as you're exercising, such as the importance of warm ups and cool downs, and controlling your breath as you exercise.

Warming up before you exercise and cooling down after you exercise will help your heart move gradually from resting to being active again. You can also decrease your risk of being sore or injury if you cool down and warm up. Warm ups should last at least ten minutes, loner for those who are older or who have been inactive for quite some time. Cool downs are especially important. If you discontinue exercise too quickly, your blood pressure will fall abruptly, which will be hazardous and can lead to muscle cramping. Try adding relaxing yoga poses to your routine.

Be sure you breathe regularly throughout your warmups, exercise routine, and your cool downs. Holding your breath will raise your blood pressure and cause some muscle cramping. Deep breathing that's regular will help relax you.

What Is Moderately Intense Physical Activity?

Use these simple tests in order to determine if you're reaching a moderate level of intensity. If you're easily able to carry a full conversation and perform the activity, too, then you are not working out hard enough. If you can sing and maintain a level of effort while you work out, you're most likely not working out hard enough.

If you can exchange a brief sentence while you're performing the activity, but it's not a comfortable or lengthy conversation, then your intensity level is on par.

If you're out of breath and you cannot even say a short sentence, you're most likely working too hard, especially if you need to stop to catch your breath.

Calculating Your Heart Rate

To calculate your target heart rate while you're working out, you need to know what your resting heart rate is. Resting heart rate is the amount of times your heart beats every minute while you're resting. The best time to figure this out is in the morning after you've just woken up after you slept very well, but before you get up. The average resting heart rate is between sixty and eighty beats per minute. However, for those who are physically fit, it's usually lower. In addition, your resting heart rate will rise with age.

Once you know what your resting heart rate is, you can figure out your target training heart rate. Your target heart rate will allow you to measure your initial fitness level and monitor your progress in your fitness program. You can do this by measuring your pulse while you exercise and staying in the fifty to eighty-five percent of your maximum heart rate. This range is known as your target heart rate.

It's imperative that you pace yourself while you exercise. If you're just starting a routine, then try to go for the lowest part of your target zone, fifty percent, during the first couple of weeks. Gradually, build up to the higher part of the target zone, eighty-five percent. After six months of regularly exercising, you might be able to exercise comfortably up to eight-five percent of your maximum heart rate. However, you won't need to exercise that hard in order to stay in shape.

Now that you know how to exercise properly to lower your blood pressure and lose weight let's talk about how to manage your stress naturally in order to lower your blood pressure.

Chapter Five – Managing Stress to Naturally Lower Blood Pressure

Stress affects your body in so many different ways, hypertension being one of them.

Additional to the emotional distress that you're

feeling when you're faced with a traumatic circumstance, your body reacts by releasing adrenaline and cortisol, the stress hormones, into your bloodstream. These hormones prepare your body for that fight or flight response by making your blood vessels constrict, your heart rate increase, and flows blood to your extremities. The constriction of the blood vessels and the increase in your heart rate raises your blood pressure temporarily. When the stress reaction goes away, your blood pressure should return to its pre-stress state. This is known as situational stress, and its side effects are typically brief and vanish when the stressful occasion has been resolved.

The fight or flight response is a valuable

reaction when you're faced with true danger that you can handle by fleeing or confronting the event. However, the modern world has many stressful events that we are not able to handle with those two options. Chronic stress causes the body to go into high gear on and off for days or weeks, which causes some serious problems.

Here are some ways that you can help manage your chronic stress.

1. Give yourself enough time to get everything done. Time management will work wonders for reducing your stress levels. Don't try to pack too much into every single moment throughout your day.

2. Learn to say no and don't over promise. Reduce your amount of rigidity by having a shorter list of things to do. This might require that you have to reevaluate your priorities and make some difficult choices, but everyone has to learn within their manageable limits.

3. You are not able to control the outside events that happen in your life, but you can change how you react to them. Try to learn to accept the things that you are

not able to change. You don't need to
solve all of your life's problems.

4. Think about problems that are under
    your control and make a plan to resolve
    them. You could talk to your boss about
    the problems you're having at work, talk
    to your neighbor if their dog is barking
    in the middle of the night, or get some
    help when you have too much to do.

5. Know your stress triggers. Think ahead
    about what might upset you. Certain
    situations can be avoided. For example,
    stop driving during rush hour and start
    avoiding those who seem to bother you.

6. Relaxing is imperative, even if you're
    busy. Take fifteen to twenty minutes
    every day to sit quietly, breathe deeply,
    and think of a peaceful image.

7. Spend some time developing nurturing
    and supportive relationships. Everyone
    needs support and encouragement every
    now and again. Invest your time and
    effort into developing relationships that

build character and foster your personal growth.

8. Give yourself the gift of maintaining your emotional health. Engage in physical activity on a regular basis. Do what you enjoy, such as swimming, walking, riding, biking, or jogging to get the big muscles in your body working. Letting go of the tension will make you feel better.

9. Limit the amount of alcohol you drink, quit smoking, and stop overeating.

10. Relax for short period throughout your day, at night, and on the weekends to help lower your blood pressure. Another good stress buster is physical activity.

11. Practice some gratitude. Change how you react to a difficult situation by focusing on the positive rather than the negative. Expression gratitude to those around you can boost your level of positivity about life and reduce your stressful thoughts.

12. Know what brings you pleasure and figure out ways to enjoy that experience. Perhaps you enjoy volunteering or cooking your favorite foods. By taking the time to not only participate in these activities but to intentionally enjoy them you can build a satisfying life rather than hurrying through those relaxing activities at a stressful pace.

Biofeedback

Biofeedback is a method that utilizes the mind to control the body's functions that normally regulates itself automatically, such as muscle tension, skin temperature, blood pressure, and heart rate.

When you first learn this technique, you'll have sensors that are attached to your body and a monitoring device. This will provide you with instant feedback on your body's functions, such as your skin temperature. Your instructor will then teach you how to monitor and how to control these functions. The results will be displayed on the monitor as you learn how to control that specific function. The monitor will beep or flash when you've achieved your desired bodily change, such as increasing your muscle tension or lowering your blood pressure.

There are two forms of biofeedback, which are EMG and peripheral temperature biofeedback. EMG stands for electromyography and is the type that uses a device to measure the muscle tension as you practice some relaxing techniques, such as meditation, visualization or progress muscle relaxation. Peripheral temperature is the type where a device is hooked to your hands and you try to increase your skin temperature, often through guided imagery or visualization.

Learning this technique requires sessions in a lab or another setting where there is an instructor. Most people have success with this technique by the time they complete twelve sessions. Home feedback units are available, too. With practice, most people can learn to influence their blood flow without the help of the monitor.

Now that you know how to reduce your stress to lower your blood pressure let's take a look at some natural remedies for high blood pressure.

Chapter Six – Natural Remedies for High Blood Pressure

While many natural remedies out there are not as effective as they tout, the natural remedies you find in this chapter have been scientifically proven to work.

Herbs

If you talk to any herbalist out there, they will tell you that taking the herbs you find in this chapter will help you lower your blood pressure.

Basil

This is a scrumptious herb that goes well with many different foods. It can also help you lower your blood pressure. It's been demonstrated that basil extract lowers blood pressure, but only briefly. Adding fresh basil to your diet certainly won't hurt, though. Keep a small pot of the herb in your kitchen garden and add the fresh leaves to your soups, pastas, casseroles, and salads.

Cinnamon

Cinnamon is another delicious seasoning that requires very little effort to add into your daily diet, and it can bring your hypertension under control. Consuming cinnamon on a daily basis has shown to lower blood pressure in those who have diabetes. Add more cinnamon to your diet by sprinkling it on your breakfast cereals, in your coffee, and in your oatmeal. At dinner, you can add cinnamon to curries, stir-fries, and stews.

Cardamom

Cardamom is a seasoning that is found in Indian and it's often used in foods in South Asia. Studies conducted where participants were given powdered cardamom daily for a few months saw a significant reduction in their hypertension. You can include cardamom in rubs, stews, soups, and baked goods for a special flavor.

Flaxseed

Rich in omega-3 fatty acids, flaxseed is able to lower blood pressure a great deal. Flaxseed might protect against atherosclerotic cardiovascular disease by lowering the serum cholesterol, acting as an antioxidant, and improving glucose tolerance. You can purchase numerous products that have flaxseed in them, but a better bet is to purchase the ground flax seed or grind it yourself in a coffee grinder and add it to home cooked meals. The best part about this seed is that it can be stirred into almost any dish, from smoothies to soups to baked goods. Store it in your freezer so it retains its optimum potency.

Garlic

This is a pungent seasoning that can do more than just flavor your food and give you garlic breath. Garlic has the capability to lower blood pressure because it causes the blood vessels to dilate and relax. This allows the blood to flow freely and reduces your blood pressure. You can add fresh garlic to many different recipes. If the flavor is just too strong for your taste, then try roasting it first. If you just can't eat it, you can always take it in a supplement form.

Ginger

Ginger might help control your hypertension because it's been shown to improve blood circulation and relax the muscles around the blood vessels. Commonly used in Asian cuisine, this is a versatile ingredient that can be used in beverages and sweets, too. Mince, chop, or grate some into your soups, stir-fries, vegetable and noodle dishes, or add it to a dessert or tea for a refreshing flavor.

Hawthorn

Hawthorn has long been an herbal remedy for hypertension in traditional Chinese medicine. Decoctions of this herb seem to have a ton of benefits for your heart, such as reducing hypertension, preventing clots, and increasing blood circulation. You can take this herb as a pill, a tea, or a liquid extract.

Celery Seed

This herb is commonly used to flavor stews, soups, casseroles, and other savory dishes. It's been long used to treat hypertension in China, but studies show that it can be effective, too. You can use the seeds to lower your blood pressure, and you can also use the juice or the entire plant. Celery is a diuretic, which explains why it's effective in lowering blood pressure.

French Lavender

The beautiful scent of this flower is not the only useful aspect. The oil from this flower has been used as an ingredient in order to induce relaxation. The herb also has the capability to lower blood pressure. While not many people think to use this as a culinary herb, you can use it in baked goods, and the leaves can be used the same way rosemary would be used.

Cat's Claw

This is an herbal medicine that's been used in traditional Chinese medicine to treat hypertension and neurological conditions for thousands of years. Studies have shown that, as a treatment for hypertension, cat's claw reduces blood pressure through acting on the calcium channels in the cells. You can get this herb in supplement form in numerous health food stores.

Power Foods

While adding beneficial herbs to your diet is an excellent choice, you might also want to add some beneficial staple foods to your diet, too. If you like any of the foods mentioned in this section, try eating one of them every day in order to boost the health benefits.

Beetroot

Nitrites and nitrates are compounds that play a huge part in the body's metabolic system. The influence they have on your body are a little confusing, but it's worth understanding if you have a blood pressure problem.

Most people believe that these components are unnatural, but that's not really the case. They are commonly added to your foods as preservatives, but they are naturally produced by your body for saliva. Nitrites and nitrates can be converted into nitrosamines or nitric oxide, the latter being the beneficial compound.

Nitrosamines are created with the nitrites are exposed to very high temperatures. Think of frying them in preservative-loaded bacon or the nitrites found in cigarettes. Most of these will increase your risk for cancer.

However, nitric oxide is a signaling molecule that's usually beneficial to your health. It gives a signal to the cells in the arteries to soften and relax. This action improves vasodilation, which helps reduce hypertension.

For this reason, nitrate-rich foods that aren't exposed to high heat are beneficial because they turn into nitric oxide. What most don't know is vegetable are a large source of nitrates in the human diet.

Beetroot is the best out of all the vegetables that contain nitrate, with most of the research being focused on the juice. So if you want to lessen your hypertension, try drinking some beetroot juice every day.

Fish Oil

Fish oil is the natural fatty acids that are found in specific fish species. These fatty acids are very beneficial to the human cardiovascular health. Numerous trials and reviews found that fish-oil supplementation is an effective treatment for high blood pressure. Yet, benefits are only seen in those who have hypertension already.

The mechanism is not clear, but most researchers believe it has to do with the omega-6 and omega-3 fatty acid ratios. Essentially, having a greater quantity of omega-3 fats in your diet is better for your heart.

Fish oil supplements are an affordable and effective treatment for hypertension and they are just as good as adding oily fish t your diet. If you have access to fatty fish, such as salmon and tuna, then two to three servings a week will provide you with benefits.

Almonds and Cashews

Tree nuts are linked with numerous health benefits. They should not be confused with peanuts, which come from the ground. Cashews and almonds stand above the rest when it comes to metabolic health benefits, such as hypertension.

What makes them so wonderful is their magnesium content. Magnesium is an essential mineral that is involved in over three hundred processes throughout the body. A lack of this mineral in your diet is associated with hypertension. Replacing that lack in the body by adding magnesium-rich foods to the diet has shown to greatly reduce hypertension.

The current recommended amount of magnesium is 310 to 410mg. One cup of cashews or almonds will provide you with 360mg.

Kale

Kale is a new superfood that is comparable to spinach. It's loaded with tons of minerals, vitamins, antioxidants, and other compounds that are known to prevent and help cure diseases.

However, the reason it can reduce hypertension is because it has a unique nutrition profile. It's rich in vitamin C, magnesium, and potassium, all of which can lower high blood pressure. Most people do not consume enough potassium, but adding kale to your diet can change that.

Turmeric

Turmeric is a very popular Indian spice added to curries. For thousands of years, Indians have not only used this spice in their cooking, but also as a medicinal herb.

Turmeric's medicinal properties have only been recently confirmed by researchers. The main active ingredient in this spice is curcumin, which has some powerful anti-inflammatory effects in the body.

The benefits that curcumin has on your blood pressure and blood flow are believed to be due to nitric oxide, similar to the beetroot that was mentioned earlier. Supplementing with curcumin has shown to help circulate nitric oxide, in some cases by as much as forty percent in four weeks.

However, there is a problem with curcumin; people are bad at absorbing it. To reap the benefits of curcumin, you need to pair it with black pepper. Black pepper has piperine, which boosts curcumin absorption by two thousand percent.

Green Tea

Green tea is from the Asian region and is loaded with tons of powerful antioxidants and compounds. The reason tea, green tea specifically, is so beneficial is due to its polyphenols. One of them is known as catechin, which has been shown to improve hypertension. Like curcumin and beetroot, the mechanism has to do with nitric oxide.

Two cups a day will increase your arterial diameter by up to forty percent. Wider and relaxed blood vessels will increase your blood flow, which reduces the pressure. It's not a surprise, then, that those who regularly drink green tea have a thirty-one percent less risk of developing cardiovascular disease.

Vitamins and Minerals

There are three vitamins or minerals that are known to lower blood pressure levels and these are potassium, magnesium, and calcium.

Potassium

Having a normal level of potassium in your body is imperative for muscle function, which also includes relaxing the walls of the blood vessels. This will help combat hypertension and protect against muscle cramping. Normal potassium levels are imperative for the conduction of electrical signals to your heart and nervous system. This will protect against irregular heartbeat.

Potassium is found in numerous different foods such as apricots, prunes, lima beans, and sweet potatoes. However, food might not be enough to keep your potassium levels high if you're taking a diuretic for blood pressure, such as hydrochlorothiazide. These can cause potassium to be leached from your body through urination, which lowers your levels considerably. If you are taking a diuretic for your cardiovascular disease, then you need to supplement with potassium.

Magnesium

This mineral helps regulate many different body systems, including your blood glucose levels, blood pressure, and your muscle and nerve function. You need magnesium in order to help your blood vessels relax, and for energy production, transporting calcium and potassium, and bone development. Just like potassium, too much can get lost in the urine when you are taking a diuretic, which leads to low levels.

A deficiency in this mineral is rare, so you should focus on getting it from foods, such as leafy green vegetables, legumes, and whole grains.

Calcium

Calcium is imperative for healthy blood pressure due to it helping blood vessel relax and tighten as they need to. It's crucial for having healthy bones and releasing hormones and enzymes that you need for your bodily functions. You should be consuming it naturally in dairy products, fish that have bones, and dark, leafy greens.

Conclusion

Remember, you need to monitor your blood pressure to make sure that your supplements and the changes you're making in your life are working. Now, they won't work overnight. Most of these changes have to be made and stuck with for at least three months before you know whether they are working or not. Most people will see subtle changes earlier than ninety days, but you have to give your body time to adjust.

I hope you enjoyed the information you found in this book. Remember, when in doubt, seek a medical provider's advice.

If you enjoyed what you found, please leave a review at your online eBook retailer's website.

Thank you for reading!

BEFORE YOU GO

If you liked this book you may like these other books from Lee Douglas

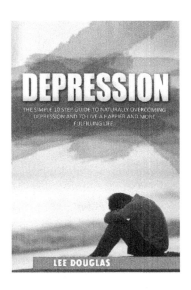

>>Check out more books by Lee Douglas<<

Free Gift

As Promised Here Is Your Guide To Managing Stress: Discover The Simple Solutions to Live A Stress Free Life.

GET YOUR COPY HERE

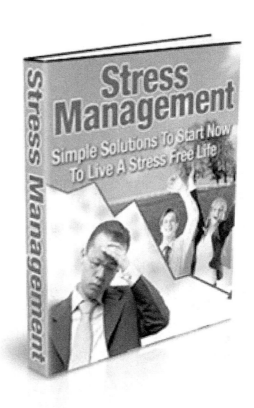

LEARN HOW TO MANAGE YOUR STRESS

Stress can take a huge chunk of your time, energy, and health. Not only your personal relationships suffer, but so as your career and total wellness. Are you struggling from stress? This book explains the true definition of stress, the symptoms and the right way to cure it. Moreover, the book gives tactical strategies to decrease your stress and increase living a happier and healthier life.

If You Want Free Best Selling Kindle Books Delivered Straight To Your Inbox

JOIN OUR FREE KINDLE BOOK CLUB!

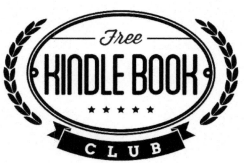

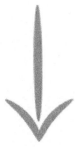

<u>CLICK HERE</u>

Finally, if you enjoyed this book, then I'd like to ask you for a favor, would you be kind enough to leave a review for this book on Amazon? It'd be greatly appreciated!

Thank you and good luck! ☺